Contents

powered by:

exclusive yoga
coaching
www.yomga.com

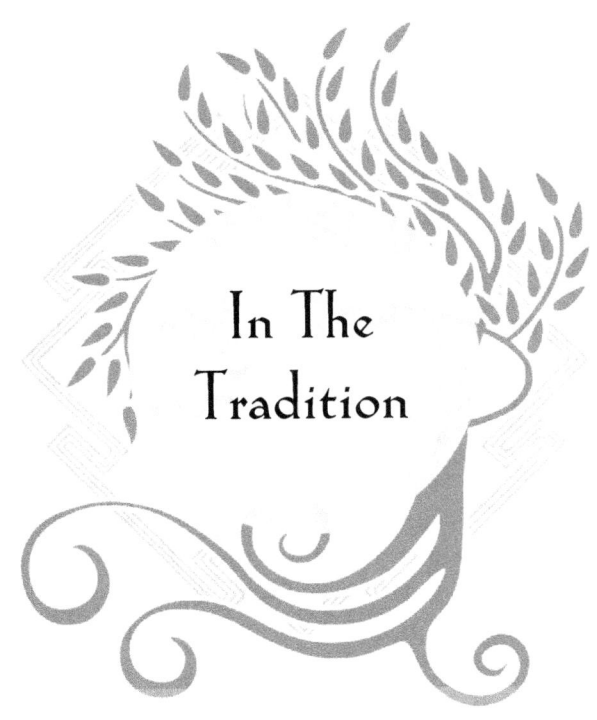

In The
Tradition

Tradition

The author of this book is not a licensed medical doctor, psychologists, psychotherapist or physiotherapist. The author is simply a student of the art of Yoga who wishes to disseminate its teachings; at the heart of which is the desire to serve others. Throughout life's journey, the author has acquired numerous insight from challenges and lessons and considers it imperative to the subservient nature of the practice of Yoga to share the lessons which have been drawn from those experiences.

In the tradition of her teachers, she continues the dissemination of knowledge based on personal experiences by only teaching what she has practiced. As such, it is advised that those who are in need of professional medical or psychological advice should consult certified professionals in those areas and not rely solely on the provisions of this book. Also, before beginning any physical practice, it is essential that you check with your medical doctor. Indeed, the whole premise of this book is the development and maintenance of self-care through nourishment of the mind, body and soul.

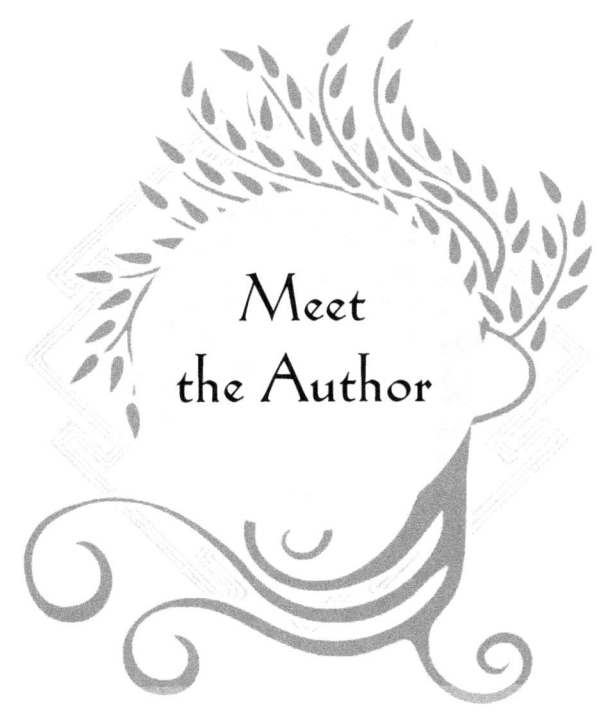

Meet
the Author

About the Author

With over a decade of experience in assisting various management teams Janaki (Janine) knows how rewarding, yet demanding, this position can be. Since the beginning of her practice, she has intentionally sought to integrate the theory and practice of Yoga into her daily life; and as such, she literally lives what she teaches. From her practices, it is relatively apparent that those ancient practices greatly increase the quality of life one experiences in today's modern society.

Intentional about following her dreams and finding her purpose, Janaki journeyed to India where she became fully engaged in the art. From those experiences she sought to educate the wider society about Yoga and refute the presentation of it being confined to an art which is inaccessible and sportive. With the benefits which Janaki experienced in her daily life, she sought it necessary to spread the well-being which Yoga could potentially bring to the world; and became certified as a 500 hour Yoga teacher. From the beginning of her yogic path, it was her aim to bring relaxation, peace of mind and overall well-being to her students, knowing that some things, simply cannot be bought.

Together with her partner she currently teaches under the formation of Yogarten, Art, Yoga and Personal development. Yogarten takes high performers on a journey to a new level that promises and delivers a better quality of life by using the ancient wisdom of Art and Yoga, in combination with personal development.

Acknowledgments

I would like to take this opportunity to thank all Yogis and Yoga teachers who have practiced and sought it necessary to keep this beautiful teaching alive today. It is only through their practice and teachings that I have found my passion and I am able to influence the betterment of the lives of others. Whatever style in whatever language is taught it serves the whole. As Swami Vishnudevanda said it so beautifully, "Unity in diversity".

Also, to my partner and best friend, a mere thank you would be quite insufficient. This man has encouraged me to practice and teach; and was also quite instrumental in helping me to spread Yoga throughout the world.

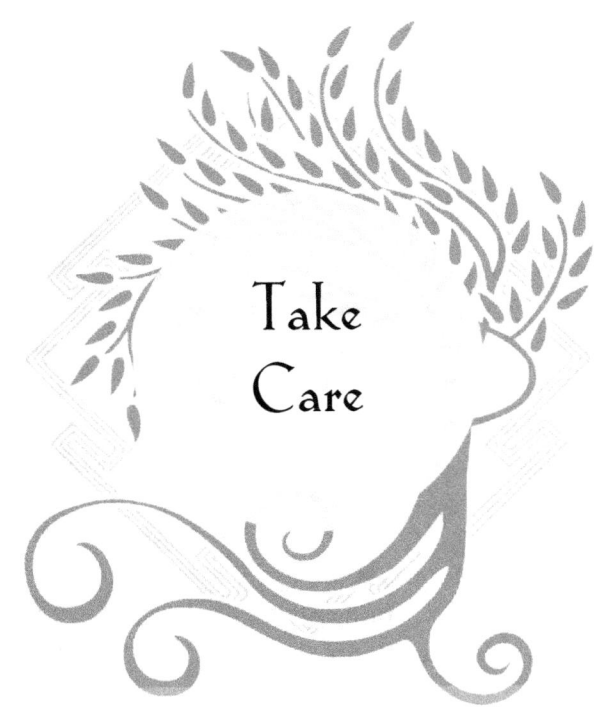

Take
Care

Introduction

Learn to Take Care of Yourself

"We are placing our attention on external objects often not realizing that we only have one body to live in and one life to live"

There is no doubt that we place most if not all of our attention on external objects and mere "things", not realizing that we only have one life to live and one body to live it in. In light of this relentless drive to achieve what we perceive as success, we often fail to realize that, in comparison to others we actually lead a comfortable life where our needs are actually met and exceeded. However, we still become consumed by the dream house and car, and avidly pursue them to the detriment of ourselves. "How do we do this you many ask?", well, to start, we constantly throw ourselves at less than desirable situations which are almost always stressful for the attainment of the desired goals.

We focus on things like work, building and sustaining a career, traveling, enduring pollution and constantly keep ourselves moving. Our days are planned down to every hour and even our sleep time is scheduled. Vacation and fun with family and friends is rarely ever spontaneous and is forced to fit in our already packed itinerary. Think about it, our minds are forced to keep up with this modern "life style" which is wreaking havoc on our mind, body and soul.

We find the time to take care of our cars, the house, our job, family and friends; but when it comes to taking care of ourselves we don't see it as a necessary investment, we come up with the most mind-boggling excuses. Think about this scenario for instance: The last time you were sick and told to rest at home, even if you did not go to work, what did you stay home and do? Did you rest?

Often times, it takes a significant life event or the occurrence of a serious health issue to force us to slow down and reconsider our priorities. However, this new found perspective is often short- lived, and once the symptom which is the driving force of our motivation to change disappears, we fall back into our most familiar patterns; completely forgetting our new intentions. You see, that is the difficulty with change many individuals experience, it is new and unfamiliar; and so we run right back to the very thing that forced us to consider an alternative perspective because it is all we know.

In general, we are always striving for more, more luxury, convenience, a nicer car and clothes, the latest phone, popular shoes and accessories; all while neglecting our mind, body and soul. We place all of our focus and energy on the acquisition of external objects, instead of making our lives better from the inside out. Believe it or not, no luxury house, expensive car or designer clothing can give you inner peace. It is time for us to realize that peace of mind and happiness cannot be bought, those things can only be achieved when we take complete responsibility for our mind and body. Yoga has the ability to provide us with balance, purifies and strengthens the body, mind and soul. We should take care of ourselves while we can and should be able to find happiness within. It is essential to note that no technology can truly control our emotions and imaginations, this is an innate power which only our bodies can possess.

Stars Know That Yoga is not Only for The Body

"Do practice while you can, you will need it when you can't."
- Krishna Das

The number of stars that avidly engage in the practice of Yoga when they are facing challenges is quite surprising. Jennifer Aniston, for example, claims that the practice keeps her in check and is her go-to practice when she needs to prepare physically and mentally for anything. Forty-one year old Gwyneth Paltrow has been quoted to have said of Yoga, "It's not just during the hours that I'm practicing. It's about how it filters through into the rest of my life. It makes all the other bullshit disappear."

What we are witnessing here is first hand benefit of Yoga on the mind. There is no doubt that both of these women are in good shape, but credit must be given to the Asanas and other practices which they incorporate in their everyday lives.

Yoga is a Private Non-Competitive Practice

"Yoga is for you alone and should be a wholesome experience"

I started Yoga because of three reasons: My back problems from sitting a day long in front of the computer, because I felt stressed and worn out from the challenges of my job and because I had the fear that my bum would one day look exactly like my office chair. My health and mind were suffering because of my daily choices and I decided that a drastic and purposeful change was needed. Fully motivated, I joined a public Yoga class in a gym, however, this wasn't as easy as I initially perceived it to be. That day, the only reason why I finished the class was because I was always determined to complete whatever I started. My body felt very stiff, I couldn't relax at all and I felt as though I had been in a car accident from the way my body ached.

I was very confused as I expected Yoga to be very relaxing and centering, yet I did not feel that way. So, I decided to go on an exploratory journey, I purchased books and DVD's and started to practice at home. I then attended another class in which I was able to keep up, but it still came across as quite stressful and intimidating. Regardless of those feelings, something deep within caused me to continue on this journey.

I journeyed to India, and there I found a passionate and patient teacher who taught small groups in a relaxing, fun and non-competitive way. I integrated those practices in my life and work and witnesses awesome results overtime. Those teaching fused the operations of my mind and body, explained its functions and reactions; and then it hit me, why is this not taught in school? I became enthused by the art and threw myself at it wholeheartedly, not long after I returned to India to deepen my studies and later pursued an advanced Yoga teacher certification in the Bahamas.

I opened my own Yoga Studio next to my "job" as I wanted to share the benefits I experienced with others. Teaching became my passion, my life and my livelihood. From the beginning it was my intention to keep the classes small and private to create a wholesome experience for the students. Philosophy, breathing exercises and Asanas were mainly focused on in the sessions. As the classes were small they became sort of personal which allowed my students to share their life challenges and nourished discussions on how Yoga had changed them. Adapted Asana classes, guided meditations and a map for a Yogic lifestyle developed for the students.

Asanas are Only One Small Part of Yoga

"Yoga was developed to be integrated in the daily life"

Someone might have suggested to you that you should start practicing Yoga, but that definitely downplays the intensity and determination necessary to stay afloat with such a practice. When we search for Yoga on the internet or in magazines, we will come upon stunning images of people hot bodies carrying out different technicalities of artistic poses, breathing exercises and the like. This has caused us to consider Yoga to be just a mere physical practice (Asana), but Yoga goes beyond the physical body and channels the mind. What most people don't understand, and perhaps I was initially of that misconception, is that Asanas are only a small part of Yoga.

Yoga is deeply philosophical and when understood in its entirety, it may be beneficially integrated into the daily life. This is exemplified as in the old scriptures where reference is made to householders (Grihastha). Housholder literally means "being in and occupied with home, family". There is no doubt that the meaning of householder has evolved over time, but the point is that individuals will always be busy and have a limited amount of time with regard to other obligations. This further makes the point that Yoga should become more of a lifestyle and not merely considered a practice in the form of Asanas.

Patanjali Maharishi, one of the greatest psychologist of all time recorded the Yoga Sutras down about 2000 years ago. This is a method of self-inquiry that takes the individual through personal changes, in a step -by -step manner. His second sutra states, "Yoga is restraining the activities of the mind". In his scriptures Patanjali writes on how the mind works, he mostly he mentions Asana as on limb, but in this context it is merely for sitting. Hatha Yoga is purposed to "purify" the whole body. The human mind and the human body has not changed much since the time of those writings, as such, Yoga offers the chance to change and improve the condition of your mind, body and soul.

Embrace the Yogic Lifestyle

"Tips and tools how you can improve your life"

This book will offer you tips and tools on how you can improve your life with the implementation of the practice of Yoga in your daily life with minimum time and effort. I will not tell you that you will be happier and healthier if you bend yourself into a pretzel shape, that a pose is easy and that you only need to breathe and it will come, that you should take two hours out of every day to practice, or that you should sit in a meditative state for hours and pretend that you are finding inner-peace and in a blissful place when you are simply planning tomorrow's presentation. What this book offers is tips which can help you to transform your life for the better with minimum time and effort.

Therefore the book is divided into 5 chapters:

1. We will create time for your practice. Chapter 1 :The time is now
2. You will learn to see and feel what you need not what you should and have to do: Chapter 2: What do you need? Connecting to your Body
3. Nobody in the history have been calmed down, by being told to calm down. Learn how to relax.. Chapter 3: Plug out to plug in.

4. Asana Basics are explained and you will learn to sequence them according to your needs. Chapter 4: Let's get physical! Love what you got, start where you are
5. You will have a road map to start living a Yogic lifestyle. Chapter 5: Yoga to go and go to

There is a Reason Why Yoga is Here

"It is your journey and Yoga can be a rich guide that shows the way."

The ancient wisdom and practice of Yoga has been around for more than two centuries, and I am sure that we need its teachings more than ever in the 21st Century. I also believe that there is a reason why you are picking up this book today, maybe you want to live healthier, be happier and content, be more successful, or even want to learn more about yourself. Whatever your motivation is, simply be open minded and ready to explore. It is your journey and Yoga can be a rich guide that shows the way.

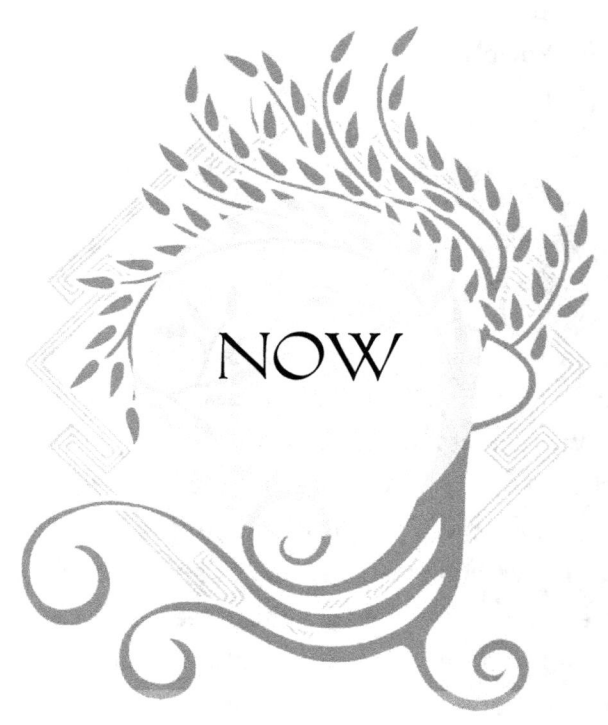

NOW

Chapter 1: The Time is Now!

Yoga Creates Time

"A clear mind is like an updated GPS having a clear goal not an obstacle"

When the mind is still we can see clearly. Consider this analogy, when you place some mud in a glass of clean water and stir it, sooner than later the water will become extremely muddy. However, if you put the glass aside and allow the mixture to stand still, you will realize that the mud will settle and eventually there will be a clear distinction between the mud and water. Even without your doing.

A clear mind is synonymous to an updated GPS keeping the aim in mind and navigating around the obstacles and not losing time by driving in the obstacles and complaining that they are there. Time cannot be created by rearranging your activities and having a tighter schedule as I am sure you have already attempted. However, having a clear mind will allow you to determine which activities are imperative for you to achieve your goals by navigating the obstacles effectively and preserving energy. The time you spend practicing Yoga becomes time you essentially save. Yoga helps you to slow down and regain clarity about your values and helps you to turn your "to do list" into a "to do what matters most list".

The Nominator of Successful People

"Where the Mind Goes, Energy Flows" - Ernest Holmes

The main consideration that sets truly successful people apart from those who never realize their dreams is their mindset. Successful people almost always focus on growth, solving problems and self-improvement; while unsuccessful people think of their abilities as fixed assets and try to avoid challenges. The truth of the matter is that the challenges which present themselves to us are just opportunity in camouflage for the determination of how badly we want to succeed. This may be further exemplified in an instance where perceiving people and things in a negative manner would lead to you missing the opportunities for growth which said individuals could provide to you.

People with a so called growth mindset, believe that with effort and perseverance, you can expand your intellect, broaden your skills, improve your character, and overcome obstacles. They see the key to getting ahead not as inherited talent or skill but hard work!

Renowned Stanford Psychologist Carol Dweck has stated that individuals who have a so-called growth mindset believe that with effort and perseverance intellect, skills and character may be broadened and improved.

Channel Your Energy

"Solutions may appear automatically"

Before joining the Yoga Teacher Training Course I often worried that I wouldn't have the time to teach. The intention to participate in the training was of course to deepen my knowledge and my practice, but I also knew that I wanted to teach in the future. At that time I still had my full- time job and the career which I had built up the last decade, and as it was a very demanding job I knew that time would be THE obstacle. This problem was solved during the course without asking for it. I learned that if I took care of my body and mind, many of the problems vanished as the solutions can be seen more easily with a clear mind. I also learned to work more efficiently with my energy. After coming back I could find support by giving away tasks from my private sector that others could do.

I made up my mind to have time and whenever I checked my work routine, my daily activities, I observed that what I thought was fixed could actually be altered. Eventually, more and more time appeared. For some it must have looked like I had worked more, but for me it did not feel that way at all. The mission was clear, my mind was made up and I got so much back from the teaching and work with my students that until today I never associated the word work with my Yoga practice and teaching.

Improve your mind through your mind

"We humans are the only ones who are able to regret the past, worry about the future or blame ourselves for what we are doing."

"The secret of conquering the tyranny of the mind is not to play the game". This is easier said than done of course. It is very ironic that us humans are the only ones who are able to regret the past, worry about the future or blame ourselves for what we are doing. This does not only makes us more likely to get ill, but also uses a high amount of energy which we could use for important tasks. Animals for example can simply find joy in their being and being present. If a dog catches a ball, it doesn't think: That was a bad catch, I could have jumped much higher, I could have landed more elegantly or what will my owner say if I bring the ball back.

No one knows exactly how the brain makes the mind. It is like the question, "What caused the Big Bang?" A common definition is: The mind is what the brain does. As humans can think about their minds, this gives hope that we are able to work on our way of thinking.

Learning to Work With the Simulator

"Mind movies can create drama excellently"

Knowing that we have a mind and that this mind creates thoughts which lead to actions give us a greater understanding of our minds. At first it might be hard to see the mind, because the western hemisphere has been brought up by the philosopher Rene Descartes statement, " I think therefore I am". It is no wonder when many of us associate stop thinking with not being. From a Yogic point of view being is simply being. We have all experienced the joy of just being present in some form or another from engaging in activities such as witnessing a sunset to more joy-filled events such as opening presents.

To create that experience more often it is helpful to become aware of the mind. How can we see the mind when we actually associate thinking with being? To create that experience more often it is helpful to become aware of the mind. How can we see the mind when we actually associating thinking with being? Here is my favorite story that a Swami once told me:

Imagine you are sitting in a theater play. The drama has reached its peak, a big quarrel is going on, someone is going to die. The shot is fired, there is a sigh going through the audience that the character is dead. What happened to you during this dramatic scene? You are still sitting in your comfortable chair.

Maybe moved by the play, wondering what is happening next.

But you did not experience the pain or the drama directly? You simply watched it, Right? The same way you are watching a play or a movie you can watch your mind. The play or movie in the mind. With practice you can sit back in your "comfortable mind chair" and watch the scene, the drama without being involved and dramatized. Our mind is constantly conversing with itself. In our mind "movies" or "simulations" are played over and over again. Replaying past events, creating drama or fantasizing the future.

Our brain is involved in over 80 % of repetitive thinking. The only thing that these movies can do excellent is create a far more better drama. Furthermore those movies or simulations keeps us stuck in our mind and are defining the future and our behavior, they are full of limiting beliefs. If we are quite honest with ourselves most of the events never even materialize, yet we are using a lot of energy while engaging with them. These simulations do not only cause stress but pull us off the present moment. It is only the present moment that we find real happiness. Seen from an evolutionary point of view, those movies and simulations have been really important for our ancestors to compare outcomes. The simulations are also important today we need to simulate a virtual reality that it is close enough to the real thing, so that we don't walk in front of a car.

Correct the Language of Your Mind

"Watch your thoughts and you will find repetitive patterns"

1.   Rephrase negative thoughts into positive thoughts to find solutions. For example: I am worn out; I need rest, I need fresh energy.

2.   Reality check: Write down your imagined ending of a situation you are going over and over in your head. For example, telling someone that you have to cancel a long scheduled and important meeting. Compare the outcome of the situation in reality with the imagined one.

Below are two tried and tested methods of making time:

You may find time by identify vampires exercise. Let's take the time to define vampire in this context, "A vampire is person who preys ruthlessly upon others and these actions may be conscious or sub-conscious."

1.   Time Vampires

How or what is stealing you time on regular basis. Example: I had a colleague once who always found me at the coffee machine engaging me in talk for over 10 minutes whilst I had the intention to nibble on my breakfast and having 5 minutes of alone time with my coffee. My whole time was used without any outcome and   it resulted in a cold coffee and hungry me. After realizing this I changed my pattern gaining more time to recharge and nourishing myself.

2.   Energy Vampires

Who or what is stealing you energy on a daily basis? There are activities that   seem at first glance relaxing and charging, but after them you will generally feel like you have less energy than before. For example: You are in the mood to have a friendly chat with a friend and meet with her for lunch simply to have a good time. You are looking forward to simply chatting away. During the lunch it turns out that the waiter is not capable of taking an order, and brings the wrong meal. And all you are doing during this precious time which should have been for chatting is attempting to get your food. What should have been an energizing lunch turned out to be a tiring experience.

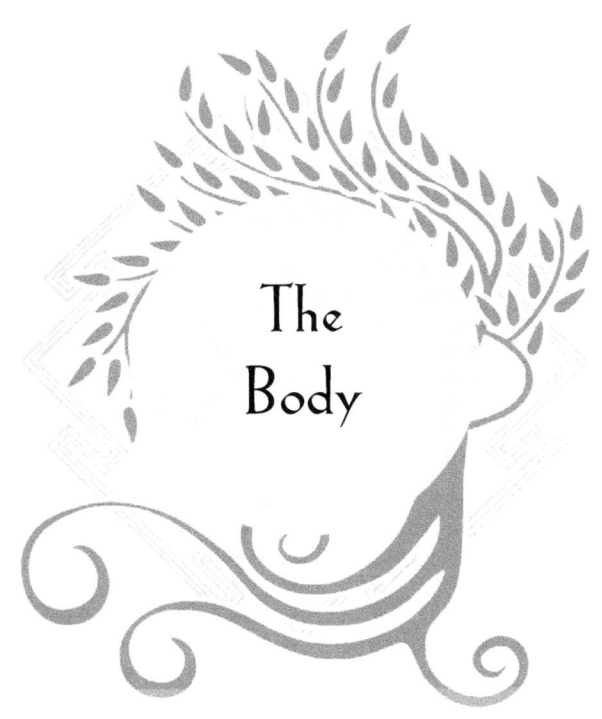

The Body

Chapter 2: Connecting to Your Body

Function on a Higher Level

"When we support our body our body supports us when we need it"

When we discover what we need life can become a lot easier. In the first chapter we learned that we have thoughts and that we are not our thoughts. Connecting back to our bodies is essential for our health, because, as mentioned before your body is the only place you can live in and spare parts are hard to find! In a way we are caring for our bodies, we wear nice clothes, put makeup on and moisturize. However, we are seldom tuned in and aware of our bodies.

When we are connected to our body, it is often because we do not feel well or that we do not look the way we would love to look. We take the functioning of our bodies for granted and when it does not function as expected, due to our lack of care, we act as though we are surprised at such an occurrence. Tuning into our bodies and intentionally finding out what it needs will not only make us happier people, but will encourage success as well. When we support our bodies they will surely return the favor and enable us to function at a higher level.

When you're not connected to your body and surrounding environment, you don't have a strong sense of direction or purpose; and you're simply existing. Also, the smallest of things can distract you and it's difficult to get anything done. When you're dealing with difficult circumstances and emotions, you may feel unbalanced and even start to shut down a little. It's all too easy to disconnect from the world when it starts to feel overwhelming.

Even When We are No Actors We Have to Play Our Part Well

"We are taking our body for granted and are just using it without being aware"

Patrick, a friend of mine is a playwright and Londoner Theater Director. I had the sincere pleasure of participating in one of his classes. When he prepares actors for their roles, he is not mainly rehearsing lines with them, but he discusses the characteristics of the role and performs exercises to connect with the body.

Additionally, he spends nearly one hour with breathing to clear the mind and create space for the role, and at least half an hour to loosen up the body. Not just relaxation, but screaming, jumping, making funny faces. He emphasizes that the participants feel and use nearly every part of the body. He says that we are taking our body for granted and are just using it without being aware. As an actor you need to be able to relate to your body at will.

Recently he started to coach people from the business world; they wanted to improve their body language and tonality; for reasons such as leading their staff better, closing more sales or being more self-secure in their negotiations. With regard to participants whose job is mainly centered around business interactions, Patrick has noticed that he has to spend a lot more time with them to bring them to a sense of self; this is because they focus mainly on their brain and less on their bodies.

Stress: The Cause of Every Illness

"Working on the source and not the symptoms"

One of my students started to do Yoga because her doctor recommended it for a problem in her digestive tract. She had to take pain killers whenever the symptoms showed up. During the class we started with breathing exercises, slowly learning how to direct breath into certain areas of the body. She learned to observe her body without being involved in the thoughts that came up during this experience. After a couple of weeks of practice she could detect the first signs and slowed down and relaxed more, as such painkillers where used less frequently. For over a year since then, the pain only occurs mildly and her body has improved rapidly. This has occurred by simply by shifting her awareness to her body.

A Toned Body is not Necessarily a Healthy Body

"Breath work is not witchcraft, it is exercising the nervous system"

What do we associate a healthy body with? Nowadays it is for sure a toned body, beautiful legs, smooth skin, a flat belly, a skinny physique which is more slim than round, right? Where does serious illnesses occur? They usually begin in your upper body, from an inner organ which is malfunctioning. In the event that you would remove your arms and legs for example, your body would still function quite normally. The major functions in your body are located from your hips upwards. So the question I am trying to ask is, would you rather have a broken foot or a defective liver?

More often than not, we judge a healthy body by the superficial and physical appearance as opposed to actual health and complete wellness on the inside. We all come in different shapes and sizes, and we have the ability to tap into our bodies to determine whether we are feeling well or ill, let's not conform to the mode of thinking that what appears to be good is actually so. Let us challenge ourselves to gain a deeper perception of self, instead of focusing on temporary vanity. Breathing not only connects you more to your body, it can calm your mind and increase your overall well being. Pranayama (Prana= life force yama= control) which are the yogic breathing exercises are a very important part of this wellness process. Yogis definitely knew how to breathe and over the last century this has been proven by scientists as more and more information has been circulation in relation to the ability of breathing properly to influence your health in a positive way. Your Autonomic Nervous System (ANS) regulates individual organ function and homeostasis, and for the most part is not subject to voluntary control; except for breathing! The ancient practice of Yoga uses breathing as a way to stimulate the parasympathetic nervous system. The Autonomic Nervous System is divided into two parts, namely; the Parasympathetic and Sympathetic Systems. The Parasympathetic Nervous System puts you into mode, while Sympathetic Nervous System activates the "fight or flight' response.

The two wings of the Autonomic Nervous System operate inversely, when one goes up the other comes down. The Parasympathetic Nervous System and Sympathetic Nervous System have evolved hand in hand in order to keep us alive and well. The Parasympathetic Nervous System produces a feeling or relaxation and a sense of contentment that's why it is called sometimes called the "rest and digest" system. When the Parasympathetic Nervous System is activated it is the normal resting state of your body, mind and brain. It helps you think clearly and avoids "hot-headed" actions that would harm you and others.

The Sympathetic Nervous System and its activation of multiple bodily systems helped our ancestors survive. In today's world with many stress factors and few life threads, a permanently activated Sympathetic Nervous System comes at high costs. Our immune systems may become vulnerable to colds, the flu and cause slower healing when we are injured. Possible results and side effects of this may include: irritability, feelings of faintness and an increased level of anxiety. If the sympathetic system is consistently stimulated without physical release of excess energy, the whole system becomes imbalanced, over stimulated and overloaded; leading to chronic diseases.

Connect to Your Body in Three Steps

"Calm the mind, calm the nervous system and connect to your body"

Here we will explore a three-step test on how you may reconnect to your body.

I. Tune In

In order to tune in and connect to your body it is necessary for you to collect yourself and come to a calm and centered place. This may be achieved with the help of deep abdominal breathing, as opposed to the often used fast and shallow breaths.

Deep Abdominal Breathing:

On inhalation, the belly should rise, on exhalation the belly should go in. The best way to practice that is to lie flat on a hard surface like a floor on your back but you can also sit up either on the floor or on chair.

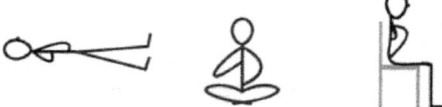

a) Place one hand on your belly and one hand on your chest. Take a deep inhalation and feel how you your belly fills, on the exhalation your belly goes in.

b) Practice this for a couple of rounds. As your lung is protected by the rib cage you won't feel much movement on your chest.

c) However, your chest will move in the opposite direction of your belly. You can transfer deep abdominal breathing in a seated posture and with a little bit of practice in your daily life.

II.   Calm Your Nervous System

Stay on the floor. When you have found your belly breath, make the inhalation as long as your exhalation. Counting: Inhaling 1, 2 , 3, 4; Exhaling 1, 2, 3, 4... And so on.

III.   Full Body Scan

Lie on your back in Savasana, your legs should be hip-width apart and your feet rolled out to your side. Your palms should face upward, with your thumbs almost touching the floor. Your chin should also be parallel to your chest. Take a couple of breaths and scan your body from foot to head and head to your foot.

Bring Breathing to Your Consciousness

"Relax when you need to"

Tune in to your body as often as you can during your busy day. Use a meeting to breathe deeply in your abdomen. Whenever I suggest this to my students, I often get a look that says: "You cannot be serious?!" However, you are breathing all day long anyways and breathing consciously does not mean that anybody notices it when you do. Even if your belly moves out more than usually nobody will notice it as nobody is looking at your belly while you are in a meeting or talking. In the event that someone is scoping out your stomach during a meeting, I'm afraid that you have much bigger problems on your hand!

Here are some other options that can help you to connect and to tune in to your body:

1. Feet on the Earth

Do you remember how relaxing a barefoot walk on the beach is? If it is not too cold walk barefooted, whether it is on the beach, in the garden or on grass. Sometimes it is important to literally connect with the earth. I find that there's something more special about actually having my feet directly on the earth rather than wearing shoes.

2. Use a Weighted Pillow

To make one yourself, all you need is a soft pillow cover that zips (a standard square throw pillow size is good; fabric should be fairly thick), a 10-pound bag of rice and some lavender if you prefer a scented pillow. Fill the pillow cover with the rice and scents. You can sit on a chair or lie on the floor and place the pillow on your lap or on your feet, or lay it across your stomach or pelvis. Sometimes it is even nice to lay it on the forehead or cover the whole face.

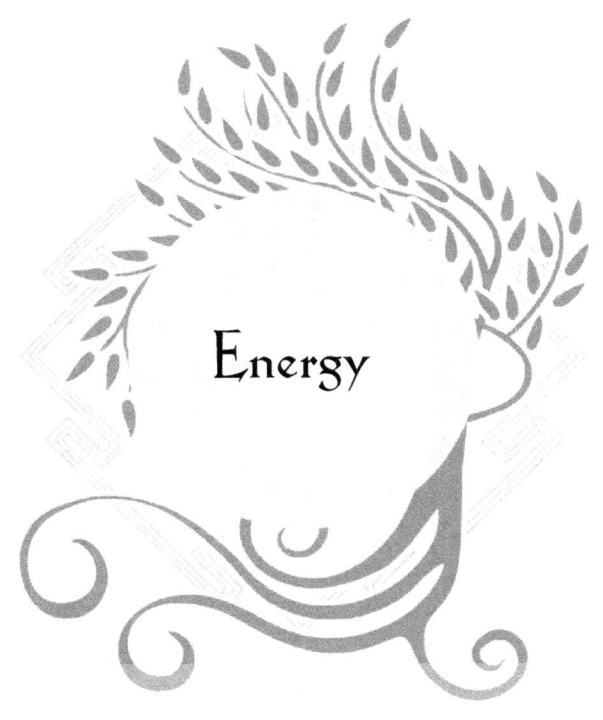

Energy

Chapter 3: Plug Out to Plug In

Allow Yourself to Relax

"Relaxation and rest is Nature's way of recharging and not being lazy"

When your phone battery is low, what do you do? You charge it! When the battery on your laptop is low, what do you do? You charge it! When you feel tired or exhausted what do you do? Work one hour more? Have a coffee? Go to the gym or go running? In our society relaxing is often associated with being lazy but relaxation and rest is Nature's way of recharging our bodies. The yogi thinks and sees often on an energetic level. When we get up in the morning we have a certain amount of energy at our disposal, this is called prana. This energy can be used the whole day or can be consumed in a moment, sometimes minutes or hours. By learning to relax, we can learn to recharge our energy and be more efficient at the tasks we need to accomplish.

We use a lot of energy subconsciously by either holding tension in our body or because of an increased stress level when our Sympathetic Nervous System is activated by bad moods, anger or even irritation. An increased stress level may have horrible consequences on our health, and to your surprise, you may even engage in some of these stress-inducing activities constantly and on a daily basis.

Energy Secret

"The state between dreaming and being awake"

What do Salvador Dali, Napoleon Bonaparte, Albert Einstein, Thomas Edison, J. F. Kennedy, Leonardo da Vinci all have in common? Except from the obvious part that they are all males and have influenced our lives in one way or another, they all napped during the days. Each of them used relaxation to dive deeper into their sub-consciousness and tap into their creative source. In the state between dreaming and waking we can recharge ourselves. What are we doing when we want to relax? Read a book, having cake, watching TV, lying in the sun? Most of us are doing something when we want to relax. Relaxation today means consuming and I don't mean necessarily spending money., either our mind is busy when we relax or our body is busy when we relax This is not true relaxation!

The True Reason Why We are All Going to a Yoga Class

"Movement for relaxation"

I saw a Yoga T-Shirt recently with the text "I am here for Savasana only" and I have to say I nearly bought one. When I go to a Yoga class I am always looking forward for this part. Savasana means corpse pose, this pose is used for relaxation, either at the beginning or the end of the class. When my students come in for class I usually ask them to lie down on their backs, then I proceed to guide them through a 1 to 2 minute relaxation, after that we start the class.

Even when we go to a Yoga class we have often have to hurry to be on time, we come from work directly or had just a brief time at home to change. By lying down even for a minute our minds can also arrive and realize that it is time for Yoga. I often end my classes with a guided 10 to 15 minutes, then we sit in it for a minute or two. With a proper relaxation at the end of an Asana class, the Asanas have the chance to be "digested" by the body as they are working not only on the muscles but on the glands, inner organs and mind as well.

When the students are opening their eyes they all have the same happy and relaxed look on their faces. One of my Yoga teachers said to a mixed international group after one class, "You know you look all the same to me now, you look all happy and content and glowing". When practicing in private we should never cut down on the final relaxation, it is better to cut down on the Asanas instead of doing only a one minute relaxation.

Me, Myself and I

"Refuge within"

For many, laying still can be quite a challenge. We have all experienced it, when we need rest and sleep the most, it is often hardest to sleep. As soon as we lie down we can hear our mind racing. I remember my first relaxation exercise many years back. I was lying on my back, asked to close my eyes and to connect to myself. My first thought was "myself what?" Either I would fall asleep immediately or I was daydreaming and 100 % involved in my thoughts. I realized that I was afraid of the silence and what would be if the silence stopped. This revelation came to me in the Ashram, we talked about the "Self", sometimes it is called "Soul" or "True Nature" in Yogic terms.

Being in touch with the Self means that there are no thoughts, no desires, no worrying just being and presence. We all have experienced this unique state at a sunset, being in nature, holding a newborn either human or animal. That is the "Self"; not the thoughts, the worries or the wants. The self or soul stands above both mind and body. Let the mind and body work, but feel that you are above them as their controlling witness.

What I have learnt during my teaching years is that there are two types of relaxers:

a)   I can find stillness through stillness
b)   I can find stillness through movement

We have to find out what works best for us and then find an appropriate relaxation technique, either before or after movement.

The Easiest and Hardest Yoga Pose

"Savasana"

In the same way that we are able to use our mind for our daily tasks, we can use our mind for relaxation. We can send messages to or muscles to contract or relax them. Under Yogic terms full relaxation is physical and mental relaxation simultaneously. In Savasana we are able to withdraw from our mind and our body. When we have created that unique space we are able to experience peace and joy and tune into our true nature. This completes the process of relaxation.

Laying Down in Savasana:

Lay on your back on a Yoga mat or blanket. Take your legs a little more than hip-width apart and let your feet turn naturally outward. Move your arms in a 45 ° angle away from your body, your palms facing up. Your thumbs should turn outwards so that your shoulder blades are touching the ground. Your chin should be parallel to your chest. You spine has its natural curve.

If you do not feel comfortable in that pose, you can either place a cushion under your head to release tension in the neck, or you can place rolled up blanket under your knees to release tension in the lower back.

In case you are not able to lay on the floor in this position you can lay on your right side. The bottom leg straight, the upper leg in an angle approx. 90 °. Your right arm is used as a pillow to support your head, your left hand is placed on the floor between bent leg and head.

Ideally, your hands and feet should not be touch anything. In winter it nice to cover yourself with a blanket. You should feel comfortable but not so comfortable that you will snooze of in couple of seconds.

When you have found your lying position make sure you can lay still for 5 to 10 minutes. Laying still simply means no movement.

Steps to Relaxation:

a) Connect to Your Body
Take a deep couple of breaths in your abdomen. Connect your mind to your body. Ask your mind to be quiet for the next couple of minutes.

b) Scan Your Body
With every inhale imagine you get fresh energy in, with every exhale you release the tension in that specific body part.

a) When you feel quite relaxed start to relax your whole body from your feet to your head. Keep saying in your mind, "I am relaxing my feet my feet are relaxed. I am relaxing my ankles, my ankles are relaxed". Move upwards to: knees, hip, belly, chest, hands, arms, shoulders, neck, head, forehead, eyes, nose, mouth, jar. You can then even move to your inner organs: liver, kidney, bladder, gall bladder, digestive system, lungs and heart. If you made it to this point without dozing off ,stay there for a couple of minutes.

b) To come out start to wiggle your toes, feet, fingers. Move your legs together and your arms over head and take a big stretch.

c) Roll to your right side, in fetal position and stay there for a couple more breaths.
d) Slowly sit up, stay seated and then get up.

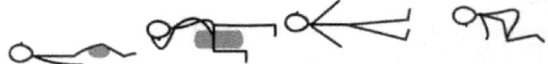

Relaxing at Will

"When lying down is no option"

Now, let's just clarify a few things, I certainly do not expect you to lay down all the time. Your co-workers certainly would not be enthused if you get up in the middle of an important meeting, excuse yourself and go and find a nice cozy place to lay down.

What we can learn is to feel the tension in our body and then relax it consciously. When you are in discussion with someone you might feel that you are making fist, biting your teeth, or simply wrinkling your forehead, this may also happen when you are working. By becoming aware of the tension you can relax it. This can literally save you energy.

When we are honest with ourselves, we can find 5 to 10 minutes every day for a relaxing break. Often we engage ourselves in energy demanding activities with the idea that we are actually relaxing. Instead, it would be wise to plug out for at least 5 minutes.

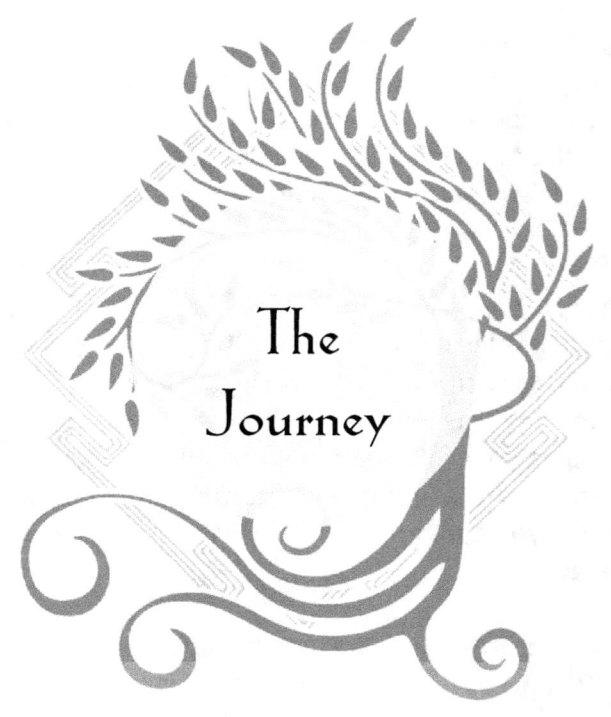

The Journey

Chapter 4: Let's get physical

Take Care of Your Safe Haven

"5 minutes and 3 square meters are enough to start!"

Practicing Yoga does not mean stepping on the mat once a week and doing Asanas it is a lifestyle in which you take responsibility for yourself. Yoga helps you to slow down and regain clarity about your values. While the ancient scriptures are sometimes hard to understand and implement into daily life, those principles are capable of integrating mind and body into an efficient and fully functional entity. Those principles create awareness and are influencing our thoughts and actions in the long run.

What I especially liked about Yoga is that there is no excuse not to practice. You cannot blame the weather because you can practice inside and outside, you do not need a membership, you do not need to pay monthly fees and to be quite honest you do not even need a mat or Yoga pants. As one of my Asana teachers used to say, "There was a time when people practiced Yoga before lululemon". Furthermore, you do not even need to have much time, sometimes even 5 minutes is enough to get you a clear mind and feeling well. Practiced regularly and not excessively, the Asanas improve your whole body and its functions.

Yoga is often sold for weight loss, calming anxiety, menopause and smooth skin however the symptoms cannot be isolated or improved through only one Asana. Let's have a look on weight loss. Some people gain weight because they eat when stressed, others are gaining weight because the thyroid is not working probably, others are gaining weight because their digestion functions are conflicted. A balanced practice can solve all those problems, through relaxation, breathing and Asanas. I like the example of the grandfather clock, when you place many of them in a room, they will all be in tact after a while. Similarly, your body consist of many parts and inner organs to create a whole system. By improving the function of your thyroid for example, all other organs benefit from it. Whatever reason you have to start you will be surprised by the effect.

Strengthen Your Strength and Weaken Your Weakness

"Yoga is the journey of the self through the self to the self"

The improvement of our strengths requires discipline and working on our weakness takes quite a bit of courage. Many of you know the story of Russell Brand. He says that Yoga improved his life to the point where he could let go of his addictions. Russell Brand states: "reality is a result of your intention and your attention". He spends nearly 2 hours on the mat practicing to keep himself on track. He also realized that the alternative of not working on himself leads to distress, addiction and a lifestyle he does not want to support anymore. From this we can understand that the things which we focus on and give our energy to essentially determines who we are and what we become. As such, it is important to be intentional about the choices which you make along your journey, with the ultimate goal being to strengthen your strengths and weaken your weaknesses.

Been There Done That Did Not Like It

"There is always a right way or an easy way"

During my travels I have always visited Yoga studios, tried new styles, gathered ideas and met awesome people. I have been melted in hot Yoga, gonged in Gong Yoga, had Yoga with life chanting, got tied up in Yoga straps, held my breath nearly for 2 minutes, stood on my head for 10 minutes. Many of those experiences widened my senses, gave me a new perspective and showed me my potential. Sometimes the hardest thing for me is to step on the mat when I feel out of balance and stressed; that is when it is hardest to connect to myself again, and that is where the work begins. The funny thing is that I always feel better and never felt worse after my personal practice.

Don't Re-invent The Wheel

"Behind every good Yoga class, there is a clear structure and purpose"

It seems that anyone who starts Yoga has to take at least 10 to 15 trial classes before a suitable style can be found for them. On top of that comes different teachers who teach the same style in a completely different way. The more people are offering Yoga and the more styles there are to choose from, the more people will practice Yoga and improve their health and their mind. It seems that every Yoga class, even when you practice the same style, seems to be different.

Yoga teachers have a lot of pressure to vary the classes as everything else in our life is new, new, new. The majority expect Yoga to be reinvented as well, but to be able to take your classes home and to practice on a regular basis a clear structure is needed. When you feel good after a Yoga class then everything is right. A good teacher does not reinvent the wheel for every class; he/she has a framework with which he/she works with. As a student it is not always easy to see this clear structure. Furthermore many students want to go to a class once or twice a week and tick it off their to do list. Asanas are meant to be practiced several times a week and the only chance to do this in our busy life is when we are able to develop a home practice.

A Safe Framework to Start and Grow Into

"Increasing the complexity"

A full practice should include: Relaxation, breath work (Pranayama), Asanas and Meditation. As we develop our own Yoga practices involving posture, breath and meditation; we can deepen our relationship with ourselves in our daily practice. Yoga classes are important to start a practice and to learn the Asanas, they are also important to have the commitment to practice Yoga regularly. From my own experience I know that starting my own Yoga practice was not easy at first, but the benefits are worth it. We so seldom spent time with ourselves (without being completely engaged in work, entertainment or other distractions) that we have to get accustomed to doing it again.

Those of you who have practiced a "fixed" series on their own know the benefits. From observing my own practice and students, I have found it helpful to use the template below. In one way it is fixed, but you can easily replace the poses according to your capabilities, knowledge and time. Once you get to know the framework, you will realize that all teachers of a full class, whether it is called Hatha or Flow, stick more or less to this framework.

Before you start:

Find a quiet room and give yourself a time frame. Turn off all sources that could disturb you such as tablets, phones and the infamous door bell. Be aware of what you want to practice today and practice in a way that recharges you and allows you to practice tomorrow. As an indicator of your progress, your breath should be calm, deep and even. The inhalation and exhalation should go through the nose only. Resting poses like Savasana, Mountain pose or Child's pose serve to assist you in finding your center again. To have a wholesome experience Asanas from every group should be practiced.

Basic template for a practice:
1. Openers
2. Pranayama
3. Warm ups
4. Sun Salutations
5. Standing Poses
6. Arm balances
7. Inversions
8. Side Bends
9. Backbends
10. Twists
11. Forward bends
12. Shoulderstand
13. Final Relaxation

1. Opening

When you have made up your mind about the days practice, choose the appropriate opener. Savasana, Seated meditation or a relaxation. Tune in and prepare yourself mentally for your practice. Give your mind time to settle down.

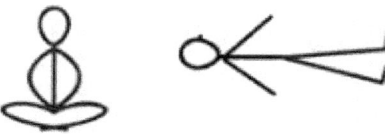

2. Pranayama

When you're new to Yoga start with deep abdominal breathing. Use the following breathing pattern. The purpose of this Pranayama exercise is to equalize the four components of the breath:

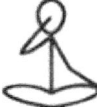 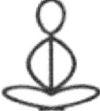

1. Inhalation (puraka)
2. Internal retention (antara-khumbaka)
3. Exhalation (rechaka)
4. External retention (bahya-khumbaka)

a) Begin with an exhale for the count of four.
b) Hold on the exhale for the count of four.
c) Inhale for the count of four.
d) Hold on the inhale for the count of four.

When you have gained more experience, do alternative nostril breathing, Anuloma Viloma or Fire breath/Shining Skull. After you have done your breathing exercise, lay down on your back and rest for a couple of minutes.

Pranayama Precaution

- Never strain the breath in Pranayama.

- If you are pregnant practice equalizing the inhale and exhale without the retentions.
- If you have high blood pressure, lung, heart, eye or ear problems it's advised not to hold the breath after the inhale.
- If you have low blood pressure it's advised not to hold the breath after the exhale.

3. Warm-Ups

Sometimes it is nice to warm up before the Sun Salutations, especially in the mornings when the body is not as flexible as in the evenings. You can do core work for greater stability in the Asanas or Lunge variations.

Core work

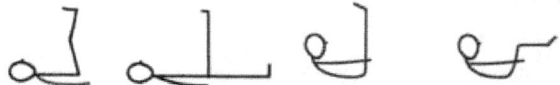

Single and double leg lifts, boat pose.

Lunge variations

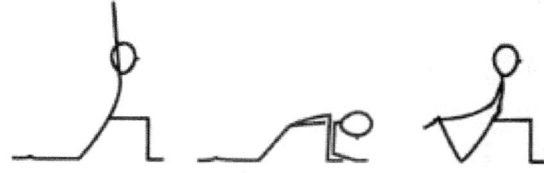

4. Sun Salutations

The Sun Salutations serve to synchronize breath and movement. All major joints are moved the spine is bent forward and backwards. Your entire body is warmed up and your circulation is increased. You can practice different styles of Sun Salutations.

Half Sun Salutations:

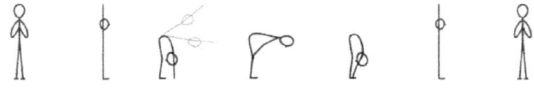

1. Stand in Tadasana hands in prayer
2. Inhale, stretch up and back, palms together, look at your thumbs.
3. Exhale, bend forward.
4. Inhale, place hand on thighs or shines and lengthen the spine.
5. Exhale, bend forward, release your neck.
6. Inhale, stretch up and back look at your thumbs.
7. Exhale, prayer.

Lunge Sun Salutations:

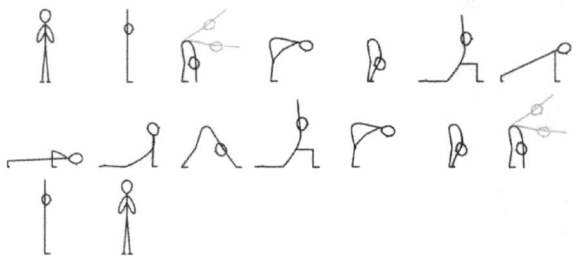

1. Stand in Tadasana hands in prayer
2. Inhale, stretch up and back, palms together, look at your thumbs.
3. Exhale, bend forward.
4. Inhale, place hand on thighs or shines and lengthen the spine.
5. Exhale, bend forward, release your neck, step on foot back.
6. Inhale, lunge hands up, palms touch, look up.
7. Exhale, come into plank pose. Inhale
8. Exhale, Chaturanga or the floor
9. Inhale, Up Dog or Cobra.
10. Exhale, Down Dog. Inhale here.
11. Exhale, foot forward.
12. Inhale, hands up.
13. Exhale, step forward.
14. Inhale, lengthen the spine.
15. Exhale, fold forward.
16. Inhale, rise, bend back, palms touch, look up.
17. Exhale prayer.

5. Standing Poses

Standing poses awaken and stabilize the entire body. They work the leg muscles and increase your ability to balance. Start with Asanas where your hip is rotated sideways, like Warrior 2, and continue with Asanas where your hip is rotated forward, like Warrior 1. This is a recommendation, not a rule. You can either do one side in a row or switch between left and right. If you need rest between the poses use Tadasana Mountain pose.

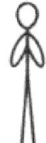

Hip rotated sideways

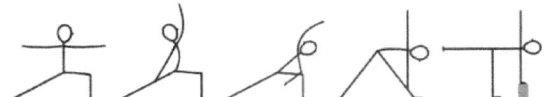

Hip rotated forward

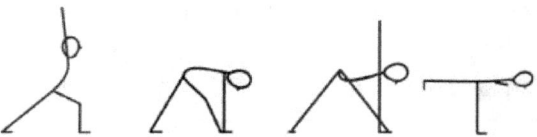

Standing balances

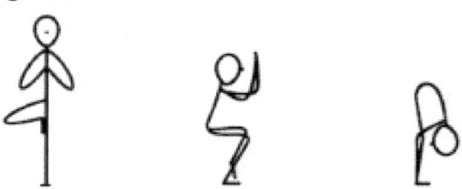

6. Arm Balances
They strengthen the arms and the upper body.
Furthermore, concentration is increased and will
power is created.

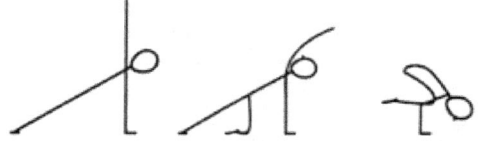

7. Inversions (practice only when you have practiced them before with a teacher)

Headstand, Forearm Balance, Handstand, Down Dog (supported)
Improves blood circulation in the upper body, legs, improves awareness and determination and blood circulation in the brain is also increased. Remember that you should always stay in child's pose after each inversion.

Handstand

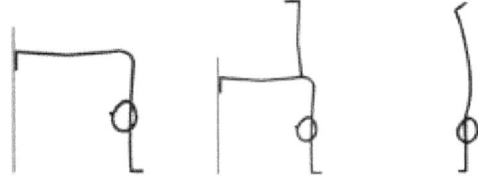

Headstand

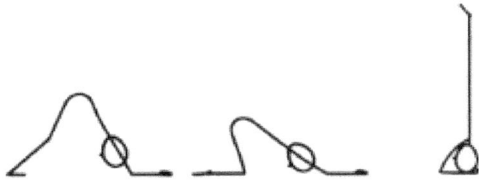

You can prepare for headstand with Dolphin pose. It prepares your shoulders for the headstand.

Forearmbalance

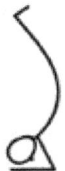

8. Side Bends
These bends prepare the body for back bends and also increase the flexibility of the spine and hip.

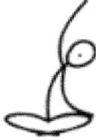 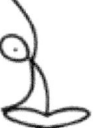

9. Back Bends
You are as young as your spine is flexible. When I started Yoga I was 80 years now I am 40, still some work for me until I am 20...
In our "forward bending" society back bends are very important to correct the hunching of the spine. They enable us to breathe deeply as they open the chest region.

Start with:
   a) Prone backbends (on the belly), like Sphinx, Cobra, Locust, Bow

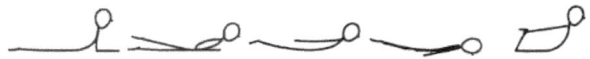

b) 2.Supine backbends (on the back), like Bridge and Wheel.

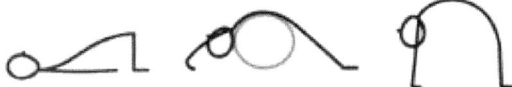

10. Twists

"Neutralize" the spine between the forward and the backwards bends.

Relax and stretch the muscles of the back as these calm the mind and the nervous system. It is also important to support deep relaxation and massage the inner organs.

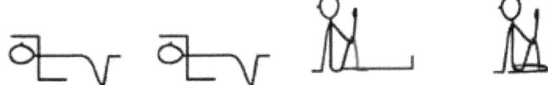

11. Forward Bends

These bends relax and stretches the muscles on the back, calms the mind and nervous system, and also gives the opportunity to turn inwards. They also promote deep relaxation and massages the inner organs

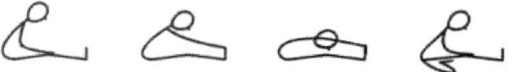

12. Shoulder Stand

Practice this pose only if you have practiced before with a teacher and if you have a healthy neck. As an alternative, you can practice legs against the wall before going in Savasana. Here the relaxation of the forward bend is deepened, it calms the nervous system and also regulates the function of the thyroid gland. Other benefits include: relaxing the heart and lowering the heart rate, elongating the nerves in the spine and relaxing head, neck and shoulders. The counter stretch for Shoulderstand is fish pose.

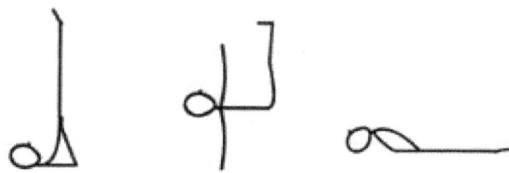

13. Final Relaxation

Set aside at least 10 - 15 minutes for your Savasana. The final relaxation gives the body time to process the information and impact of the Asanas. The unique state of mental and bodily relaxation at the same time can be experienced.

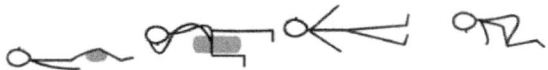

After you have completed your practice it is good to sit down for a couple of minutes for meditation.

Love What You Got, Start Where You Are

"Life is a journey not a destination"

At the beginning choose accessible Asanas that work for you and place them in the aforementioned order. You won't find gold, enlightenment or everlasting happiness when you can reach your toes and it does not make you a better person. What is important is what you learn on the way towards touching your toes. Maybe it is patience, kindness or even learning more about your thought patterns and how your mind works. I don't say this to discourage you, but when you have mastered an Asana there is always an advanced version of it, and when you mastered that one there is still the Chinese circus to compete with!

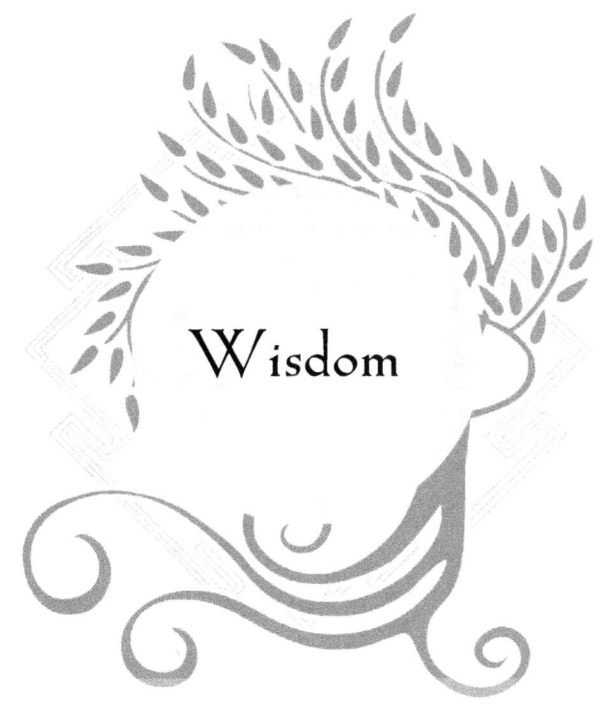

Wisdom

Chapter 5: Yoga to go and go to

You are Your Best Assets

"Invest in Yourself"

Our creativity, our uniqueness, our skills and our ability to adapt can set us apart from our competition, and from getting replaced by technology. To keep on track and be in excellent form, it is important to grow and to sustain our career. We invest in a new computer to work more efficiently, we take our cars regularly to check up on their functions, we update our apps on our mobiles, yet we seldom take time to look deeper into our habits and to find out how we function and work.

Sharpen Your Axe

"If I had six hours to cut down trees, I would spend the first three hours sharpening my axe and the last three cutting down the trees."
- Abraham Lincoln

We all know the stories of the two wood choppers and it is pretty obvious to us that the chopper who loses time to sharpening his axe will make it good later on and have a much easier task to accomplish as he had prepared for the requirement her knew was ahead. Yet it has happened to all of us that have been so consumed by our work that we forgot to take a break, to sleep, to eat or even too pee. Luckily, some functions of the body cannot be ignored and we receive a warning before the undesirable occurs.

We need to sharpen our axe as well, and prepare the tools we need to work on our mind, heart, body and habits. All great leaders had a system that was adaptable to their habits. When we read their diaries or notebooks we realize that nothing was left to accident or chance. There was a clear structure behind their day. They took time and courage to investigate their needs and wants, and from there sought to create a feasible plan that would support their habits. They also created an environment that would be supportive of those desires. They also took time to review it and adapt to it when necessary but still keeping their main goal in mind.

A Holistic System

"Mind, Body and Soul"

My search brought me to beautiful places, I
travelled with a backpack in Europe, I camped, I
searched refuge in nature and in European
Metropolitan areas, I stared at the ocean, I went to
India. I danced ballet, I hiked, I lifted weights, I
climbed the career ladder, I took care of
apprentices, I learned to speak and write in English.
We all had a time in our life when wanted to go out
and search, to search so that we could embrace
becoming something more, something greater.
What I learned during my travel is this, you cannot
run, and you certainly cannot hide from yourself as
you are on this holistic journey with your mind,
body and soul. To become my own friend was what
I essentially learned. Sometimes the criticizing and
nagging voice in our heads can be useful. I learned
to see my needs and wants and as soon as I treated
them accordingly, life not only became better and
easier; but my energy level to perform my tasks and
duties increased.

Stick to The Plan

Social media and commercials are always on the search for novelty to increase their sales figures and to strengthen their market penetration. There is a constant informative stream that tells us who you should be, what you should wear, buy and even eat. However, this intention is only to fill a global players pocket with more money, as opposed to providing a necessary need or even encouraging health habits. Many of these novelties are certainly convenient and fascinating, but the high risk of association with dis-ease is simply shocking! When we want to move around at work, instead of taking the stairs we ride the elevator; when we want to exercise more, we invest in fancy gadgets such as smart watches and then become overly stressed about not attaining the requirements set by a mere machine, as opposed to listening to our bodies which yearn for our attention.

It is totally okay as long as you create a valuable experience for yourself and is not devastated by the disappearance of those objects from your life. We can also use those objects as leverage to bring us into a certain mood, the Yoga pants to do Yoga, the new dress or suit to get the job, the bottle of Champagne to celebrate our birthday, the class of wine to close a long and hard workweek.

We define ourselves over brands and boost our self-esteem and worth through meager items such as clothing, cell phones and shoes. Having these items are totally okay as long as they bring value to our lives and we are not devastated when those of objects disappear. However, we are losing a lot of time and energy by focusing on these simple things instead of focusing on self as a whole.

5 Habits for a Happier You

"Ancient wisdom for a happy now"

Whatever diaries of successful people I have checked for habits, they truly come down to these five. Of course sometimes they are named differently or are structured more detailed. I also checked contemporary health apps, which drove me nearly crazy, come down to them. You can rename them, add one or delete one. But personally I found that I can stick to them because they are easy to remember and implement and do not give you a guilty conscience when you forgot one during the day.

To integrate Yoga into daily life the Swami and founder of the Ashram in which I studied, synthesized the ancient wisdom of Yoga into five basic principles:

1. Positive Thinking/Meditation
2. Proper Breathing
3. Proper Relaxation
4. Proper Exercise
5. Proper diet

1. Positive Thinking/Meditation

When the mind is focused and concentrated all problems, worries and thoughts will disappear. We can develop our concentration by starting to be attentive in everyday situations. Throwing the attention into whatever is being done shuts done all other thoughts and forces the mind to conform. Will power and memory is developed when we train our mind to attend only the work at hand. When we manage our time and minds well, we will come to the realization that tasks may be done accurately and in half the time.

Meditation is not something that can be taught you, already have the innate ability to shut out your thoughts. One cannot learn to meditate, in the same way one cannot learn to sleep. What we can learn is how to calm our mind and how to prepare our body for sitting. During meditation there is a constant observation of the mind. Meditation brings mental peace, and on a physical level meditation helps the processes of growth and repair.

Simple Steps to Meditation:

a) Have as separate room, or a screened up spot in a room that you can use exclusively for the purpose of meditating. Make it appealing and comfortable for yourself so that you can relax and feel peaceful. Set a specific time for your meditation so that you will get into the habit of returning your practice.

b) Focus on your breathing and breathe deeply into your abdomen, make the length of the inhalation as long as the length of the exhalation. Inhale for 3, exhale for 3.

c) Let your mind wander at first, watch your thoughts without interacting with them. If your mind does not settle down, count your breath again

d) Select an internal focal point for your mind; either between the eyebrows or at the center of your heart.

When we meditate we watch our mind from a neutral place and don't interact with our thoughts. We become a detached witness of the mind. The most important thing is to be patient with yourself. At first instance, you might be able to sit for 5 minutes, but the time will increase with a little bit of practice. I find it helpful to set a timer and sit the time I set for myself. With this method my mind does not ask itself how much time has passed yet.

2. Proper Breathing

In Yoga, breath is more than just oxygen, it is the life force through Pranayama, you use the breath to affect the constellation of energy that is your body-mind. Prana is called Chi in Chinese and Ki in Japan. We can picture the prana system similar to our nervous system. In China this map which consists of meridians is used for acupuncture. The Yogis call this system the nadis, we are supposed to have 72,000 nadis. To stay healthy, the prana has to flow. Therefore breathing exercises have been developed to facilitate these achievements. Whether you believe in Prana or not, here are some mind blowing effects of its practice:

- Improving concentration and memory
- Helping with weight loss and improved digestion
- Waking up feeling rested
- Relieving headaches, migraine
- Strengthening the immune system
- Reducing high blood pressure
- Reducing cardiovascular risk
- Reduces anxiety and depression
- Improving regulation of blood sugar levels

3. Proper Relaxation:

It is recommended that you employ the use of the relaxation options previously mentioned. However, what is most important is learning to feel tension in the body and being able to relax at will.

4. Proper Exercise:

This is the stage at which your Asana practice comes in handy. However, if you are unable to get on you mat for whatever reason; make it a point of duty to move your body intentionally. So go right ahead and take the stairs and stand up at intervals when working around a computer. The term Asana means steady pose, so every Asana should be held for some time. Yogic exercises cannot be compared to any other system. Our body is more than muscles and skin, and everybody who had a health issue with an inner organ, such as a malfunctioning thyroid, knows how it can affect everyday life and its quality.

5. Proper Diet:

Innumerable books and journals have been written on nutrition and dieting. Where on the one hand gaining access to good food has never been easier, our modern lifestyle hardly gives us time to take care of ourselves. Each and every person has to decide what a proper diet means. Regardless of whether you follow a vegetarian, vegan or Paleo diet, there still exists the possibility of eating unhealthily. Eating in a healthy and energetic way the food should have a lot of sun, water and air.

In the context of Yoga a vegetarian diet should be chosen. The Yogi should practice non-violence (Ahimsa), and by eating meat he violates that regulation (Yama). Another reason why vegetarian food is preferred is because the Yogi thinks in an energetic way. Every being is stressed when it dies;

there is no point of discussion on that subject, so by eating meat the stress hormones go into the system of the Yogi and causes imbalances in his body. When I eat this way I know that I feel lighter and cleaner, my mind is sharper, sitting still is easier, and the Asanas are more graceful. However, I also know that I can run on a Croissant, Cheese, Baguette and French Wine diet for a week and half and still practice Asanas, work, and be in a healthy mindset.

Be You, Being Yogi

"There is just one you!"

Go for a Yoga class with a teacher that supports you, meet same-minded people and get new ideas. Although the aforementioned can be greatly beneficial, it is imperative that you practice on your own and be independent in those practices. Practice, just practice for yourself and yourself alone.The experiences and trials which you gain from the journey on your mat may be used in everyday life, and I assure you that you will witness mind-boggling changes if you simply submit to the very nature of your being and embrace the process. Yoga means taking responsibility for yourself, your life is simply what you make of it.

With the methods presented in this book, you will know and feel when you pushed yourself too hard, you will know when you have improved in an area of your life, you will know when you are honest with yourself. Yoga is self-love in the most non-egoistical way. You will be more successful, see more beauty and definitely be happier. You will be able to fulfil your duties and purposes effectively and therefore contribute to the betterment of this world as only you can!

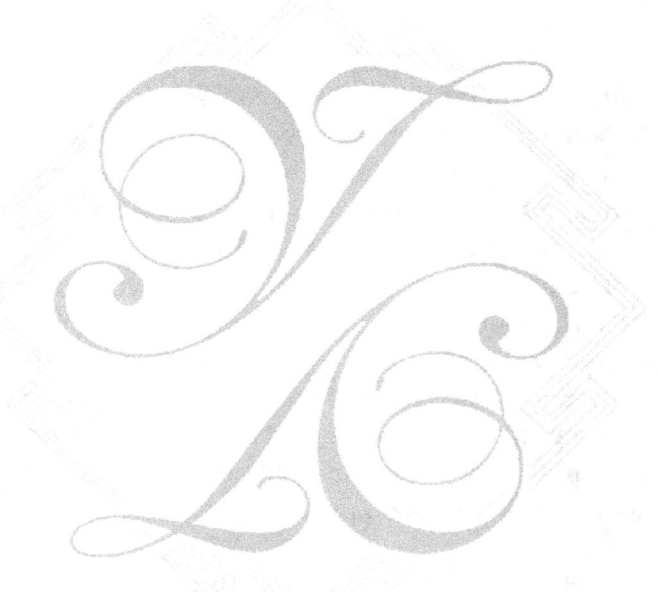

get free videos:
CODE: YYV089
info@yogarten.com